The Holistic Athlete

Alternative Therapies for Fitness and Nutrition

Table of Contents

Chapter 1. Introduction

Dive into a refreshing new perspective on fitness and nutrition in our exclusive Special Report "The Holistic Athlete: Alternative Therapies for Fitness and Nutrition". This comprehensive guide serves as your ideal companion, exploring the world of holistic health practices and their positive impact on athletic performance. From acupuncture to vegan diets, we comprehensively shed light on unique methods athletes use to enhance their fitness, manage injuries, and improve their nutritional intake. As you navigate these enriching pages, brace yourself for an enlightening journey. Sweep away preconceived notions and embrace a blend of science and nature that fuels the holistic athlete inside you, potentially revolutionizing your fitness and nutritional regime. Cheerful in its delivery and insightful in its content, this report is all set to inspire your sporting spirit and invite the change that could lead you to peak performance. Don't miss this opportunity! Get ready to explore, learn and thrive!

Chapter 2. Unraveling the Concept of Holistic Health

The world of fitness and nutrition has evolved far beyond lifting weights in the gym and the classic high-protein diet. As our lifestyles and scientific understanding have evolved, so has our approach to maintaining a healthy body. In the pursuit of optimal health and wellness, more and more individuals are looking towards holistic health – a concept that emphasizes the connection between mind, body, and spirit. Let's dig deeper into this ground-breaking approach.

2.1. Understanding Holistic Health

Holistic health or holistic medicine is, at its core, about taking the whole person into consideration - physical, psychological, social and spiritual aspects - rather than focusing purely on symptoms of illness. The aim is to strike a balance in life, leading to optimal health and wellbeing. The ethos of holistic health promotes the idea that the body can heal itself if given the appropriate tools. Those tools don't have to be purely pharmaceutical; they can include things like diet, exercise, therapy and relaxation techniques that we'll discuss in depth later in this chapter.

2.2. The Origins of Holistic Health

Holistic health practices can be traced back to ancient civilizations, including the Greeks, Egyptians, and Indians, who understood the importance of treating the whole individual rather than only a single ailment. The healing traditions of Ayurveda from India, Traditional Chinese Medicine, and various Native American healing practices are all rooted in the principle of holistic health. The modern resurgence of holistic health began in the late 20th century and continues today, integrating traditional practices with modern medical knowledge.

2.3. The Principles of Holistic Medicine

The principles that guide holistic health are fundamentally different from traditional western medicine. They revolve around the understanding that optimal health is not just the absence of disease. Below are the core principles:

1. The individual is seen as a whole — recognizing that each part of the body is interconnected and interacts with other parts to function effectively.

2. It values patient empowerment — patients play a vital role in their healing process, taking responsibility for their health and making informed decisions about their care.

3. It doesn't just focus on eradicating symptoms, but instead, it targets the root cause of the illness.

4. It emphasizes prevention and health promotion as critical for achieving optimal wellness.

2.4. The Importance of Balance in Holistic Health

Central to the holistic health philosophy is the idea of balance. This balance refers to achieving harmony among the body's systems and between the body, mind, and spirit. To present a clearer picture, consider these three elements as interconnected facets of a single entity. When one part is off-kilter, it impacts the others and thereby disrupts the overall balance. Consequently, a holistic approach aims to restore this balance through lifestyle changes, alternative therapies, and mindful practices.

2.5. Nutrition in Holistic Health

In holistic health, what you feed your body plays a crucial role in your overall wellness. The belief is that nutrition is about more than just calories or macronutrients. It's about eating wholesome, organic foods that are nutrient-dense and provide the body with the energy it needs to function optimally.

Holistic nutrition focuses on consuming a balanced diet rich in fruits, vegetables, lean proteins, whole grains, and healthy fats, with focus on local and seasonally available produce. Also, it encourages mindfulness in eating, respecting the food and understanding its importance for health and wellbeing.

2.6. Exercise and Holistic Health

Physical activity is another cornerstone of holistic health. It's not just about rigorous workouts, but rather finding movements you enjoy and that work in harmony with your body. Whether it's strength training, yoga, Pilates, walking, swimming, or hiking, it's vital to incorporate regular and varied physical activity into your daily routine. The goal is to maintain physical abilities, raise endorphins for mental health, and support a balanced metabolic state.

2.7. Mind-Body Connection in Holistic Health

The mind-body connection is a vital component of holistic health. This connection recognizes that our thoughts and attitudes can affect our physical health. Techniques such as meditation, mindfulness, yoga, and Tai Chi can help individuals manage stress and anxiety, improve their mood, and achieve a state of mental and emotional balance. These techniques can lead to a remarkable improvement in quality of life and overall wellbeing.

2.8. Holistic Health and Alternative Therapies

Alternative therapies play a significant role in holistic health. Treatments like acupuncture, chiropractic work, homeopathy, massage therapy, reiki, and naturopathy are often incorporated to complement lifestyle adjustments. The choice of therapy depends on individual needs and preferences and should ideally be undertaken under the guidance of a skilled therapist.

Holistic health is about redefining how we view health, wellness, and disease. It involves taking responsibility for our health, making beneficial lifestyle changes, and focusing on preventative healthcare. While this approach may not be the answer for all health problems, it provides an excellent foundation for maintaining health and preventing disease. It is about fostering an environment within ourselves that encourages health, rather than condoning disease. In essence, holistic health invites us to treat our bodies with respect, be mindful of our choices, and strive for a balanced life.

Chapter 3. The Athletic Body: Understanding Kinesthetics

In the pursuit of peak performance, understanding the athletic body's mechanics, or kinesthetics, is vital. Kinesthetics involves self-perception of one's movements, providing athletes with valuable insights about their athletic performance and future improvements.

3.1. Essential Principles of Kinesthetics

Kinesthetics rests on a set of principles which govern our understanding of this science. The concept of proprioception is at its core, defined as the body's intrinsic understanding of its position in space. This skill is integral to athletes, allowing them to maneuver their bodies adeptly during training or competition, regardless of whether they can visually track their movements.

Extending this fundamental aspect of kinesthetics, we touch upon the notion of balance. Balance is a critical skill for athletes across a wide swath of sporting disciplines. The sense of equilibrium in active movement and static positions aids in both power and precision, facilitating optimum execution. Training programs often incorporate specially tailored drills to hone this kinesthetic sense.

3.2. Amplifying Athletic Performance

A well-developed sense of kinesthetics can yield significant improvements in athletic performance. An in-depth comprehension of the body's capabilities and limitations can result in superior technique, precise execution, and reduce injury risk. Kinesthetics encompasses the sportsman's ability to balance, coordinate movements, and understand his bodily positions, effectively aiding in speed, force, and precision enhancement.

This acumen can be fine-tuned through practice. Activities like yoga, martial arts, and dance are advantageous in refining the body's kinesthetic senses. Each of these programs offers a unique approach towards a more harmonious body awareness, encouraging an athlete to be more conscious of their physical movements and the space they occupy.

3.3. Spacing and Body Positioning

One of the lesser-known aspects of kinesthetics, yet crucial to athletes, is the awareness of body spacing and positioning. Athletes need to possess an innate sense of how their bodies relate to their surroundings, contributing to split-second decisions and precise maneuvers during a game. Sports like football or basketball, where athletes often need to judge distances and adjust their position spontaneously, exemplify this importance.

Practices like Tai Chi and Qigong foster this sense of spatial awareness along with fostering physical coordination. Known for their measured movement sequences, these disciplines encourage awareness and mindfulness, serving as a holistic method for every athletic endeavor.

3.4. Importance of Rest and Recovery

Within the context of kinesthetics, recovery and rest play a pivotally important role. A tired athlete's kinesthetic abilities can falter, leading to reduced performance and increased injury risk. To maintain their inherent kinesthetic cognizance, athletes must focus on rest and recovery, ensuring the body and mind are equally refreshed and energized.

Athletes are encouraged to turn to practices such as meditative body scans, guided visualizations or restorative yoga to help them reconnect with their physical bodies. This not only aids in improved performances but also contributes to injury prevention and mental well-being.

3.5. Nutrition: Fueling the Kinesthetic Machine

Just like a machine operates best with the right type and amount of fuel, the athletic body also relies heavily on nutrition for optimum performance. From muscle recovery to energy provision, nutrition is the silent architect behind an athlete's success.

Nutritionists recommend a balanced diet rich in protein, complex carbohydrates, and good fats. The right mix of these macro nutrients ensures sustained energy, faster recovery times, and improved resilience in athletes.

Staying in tune with the body's fueling needs is as crucial as fine-tuning its performance. Supplements, hydration, and a personalized eating plan add invaluable elements to an athlete's lifestyle. A comprehensive nutrition plan serves not only as a fuel provider but also a recovery agent, completing the circle of kinesthetic awareness.

3.6. The Holistic Approach to The Athletic Body

In essence, kinesthetics is the science of 'body wisdom.' A true comprehension of this body-machine can offer profound insights for any sports person. Aiming to elevate our understandings from just form and performance to include awareness and integration, a holistic approach is the edge that could redefine athletic success.

Athletes are encouraged to broaden their perspectives beyond just the physical, to include elements of mental and emotional health as well. Sports psychology, nutrition, sleep science, and breath-work are some tools under this holistic approach that can significantly enhance one's athletic journey.

The understanding of kinesthetics doesn't just contribute to an athlete's performance enhancement but also instills a sense of mindfulness that transcends way beyond sports. By being truly in tune with our bodies, we can cultivate an ingrained body wisdom that nurtures us in every aspect of life, sports or otherwise.

Chapter 4. Diet and Nutrition: The Lifeline of Performance

The journey towards optimized physical performance begins with an understanding of the lifeline that feeds it: Diet and nutrition. Traditionally, athletes have tailored their diets to meet the specific demands of their sport, but as we increasingly come to understand the human body and its individual needs, the importance of a holistic perspective has become indisputable.

4.1. Energy Fuel: The Basics

Let's start by exploring the basics of nutrition. At its core, all food is broken down by our bodies into macronutrients and micronutrients. Macronutrients, namely proteins, carbohydrates, and fats, provide the fuel our bodies need to function. They support muscle growth, energy production, and cellular repair. Micronutrients, on the other hand, are the essential vitamins and minerals that we require in smaller amounts, but are crucial for optimal body function and injury prevention.

For any athlete, a balance of these nutrients is important. Carbohydrates serve as the body's primary source of energy during intensive physical activities, while proteins are needed for recovery and muscle tissue repair. Fats, particularly the unsaturated variety found in foods like avocados, nuts, and fish, are also necessary as they support cell growth and protect the body's organs.

4.2. Optimizing Performance : The Power of Antioxidants

Beyond the basic understanding of macronutrients and

micronutrients, lies the realm of antioxidants. These are compounds found in certain foods that can prevent or slow damage to cells caused by free radicals. Synthetic antioxidants can often be found in supplements, but they also occur naturally in a variety of fruits and vegetables.

For athletes, an antioxidant-rich diet may help to improve recovery times and reduce muscle damage. Foods high in Vitamin E, such as seeds, greens, and tropical fruits, along with Vitamin C rich foods like bell peppers, oranges, and strawberries are excellent choices. The rich colors in beetroot, tart cherries, and acai berries are indicative of their high anthocyanin content, which has been linked to reduced inflammation, improved blood flow, and overall better physical performance.

4.3. Personalizing Your Nutrition: The Art and Science of Nutrigenomics

Every individual is unique in their nutritional requirements. Several factors such as age, sex, genetics, the intensity of physical activity, and specific health and fitness goals will determine your optimal diet. The emerging field of nutrigenomics is proving that there isn't a 'one-size-fits-all' approach to nutrition.

Nutrigenomics focuses on understanding how food influences our genes and how individual genetic differences can affect the way we respond to nutrients (and other naturally occurring compounds) in the foods we eat. Athletes, through genetic testing, can now understanding their genotype and optimize their diets to enhance performance, boost recovery and minimize the risk of injury.

4.4. Tweaking Nutritional Intake: Carb Cycling and Intermittent Fasting

The fine-tuning of macros, alongside meal timing, can have profound effects on athletic performance. One dieting technique that's garnered attention in recent years is carb cycling. Carb cycling involves alternating between high and low carbohydrate days. On high-carb days, your body is fueled to perform high-intensity workouts, and on low-carb days, your body is more inclined to burn fat.

Similarly, intermittent fasting (IF) has gained popularity among athletes. IF is an eating pattern that includes periods of eating and fasting. It does not specify which foods to eat but rather when to eat. Evidence shows that practicing IF can reduce inflammation, improve brain health, and promote fat loss when coupled with resistance training.

It is important to note that while these approaches may work for some, they may not best suit everyone. It is advised to experiment with different dietary strategies under the guidance of a qualified professional to determine what works best for you.

4.5. Plant Power: Vegan Diets for Athletic Performance

The move towards plant-based diets has been one of the most prevalent trends in sports nutrition. Increasingly, athletes are turning to veganism for a variety of reasons, including health benefits, ethical reasons, and to reduce environmental impact.

Well-planned vegan diets can provide all the necessary

macronutrients and micronutrients required for optimal athletic performance. Key considerations for vegan athletes include ensuring adequate intake of iron, zinc, calcium, and vitamin B12, nutrients which are commonly found in animal products. These can typically be met through a variety of plant-based foods and fortified food products.

A diet rich in plants tends to be high in fiber, antioxidants, and other phytonutrients, which can provide several performance advantages. Systematic review studies have highlighted benefits including improved blood flow, better heart health, faster recovery times, and increased endurance.

4.6. Hydration: The Unsung Hero

Last but not least is the often overlooked role of hydration in athletic performance. Every cell, tissue, and organ in our body needs hydration to work properly. Athletes need to take extra care to maintain hydration levels due to the additional loss of fluid through sweat. Dehydration can significantly impair sport performance by causing decreased strength, impaired mental function, and general fatigue.

Athletes should aim to start their training sessions well-hydrated and replace any lost fluid through sweat by consuming fluid-rich foods or drinking beverages that are composed of water, a moderate amount of carbohydrates, and electrolytes.

In closing, maintaining a holistic approach to diet and nutrition can serve as a propellant to peak physical performance. The journey towards your fitness goals is very much a personalized ride; it calls for continuous education, close attention to your body's cues, and ongoing adjustments to your nutritional strategy. Remember, integral to that strategy are alternative methods of optimizing fitness that aren't only about what's on your plate, but also how your body interacts with it. Be prepared to embrace the change, envision the transformation, and feel the difference!

Chapter 5. Alternative Medicine and Athletic Performance

Alternative medicine is increasingly becoming a viable option for athletes looking to maximize their performance, recovery, and overall well-being. The efficacy of these alternative therapies varies from person to person, but they are generally used as a means to complement traditional methods of care.

5.1. Acupuncture and Athletic Performance

Acupuncture is a form of traditional Chinese medicine that has been in practice for thousands of years. It involves inserting fine needles at specific points on the body to restore balance and promote natural healing. Acupuncture is thought to stimulate the nervous system, which can help athletes increase their energy levels, improve their mental clarity and focus, and enhance their overall performance.

The application of acupuncture in sports is multifaceted. Some use it as a treatment for acute or chronic pain, others incorporate it as part of their recovery process, and there are those who utilize it to enhance their mental toughness.

Certain studies suggest that acupuncture may help to speed up muscle recovery by modifying inflammatory responses and increasing circulation. These benefits may provide athletes an advantage by reducing downtime and allowing more frequent training sessions. More research is still needed to fully understand the clinical application of acupuncture in sports, but the preliminary findings provide a promising outlook.

5.2. Chiropractic Care and Athletic Performance

Chiropractic care is another popular treatment modality used by athletes. It primarily involves manipulation of the spine to optimize neuro-musculoskeletal function. Athletes commonly suffer from musculoskeletal disorders due to intense training and competition, and chiropractic care can help to restore mobility, alleviate pain, and promote proper alignment of the body.

Chiropractors may also use other treatment modalities such as stretches, massage, and nutritional advice to achieve comprehensive care. There is a growing body of evidence showing a positive relationship between chiropractic care and athletic performance. This has resulted in increased acceptance and usage of chiropractic care among athletes.

While chiropractic care can complement traditional sports medicine, athletes should ensure they receive treatment from a well-qualified professional due to the risk of inappropriate or excessive manipulation, which could result in injury.

5.3. Herbs and Supplements

Herbs, supplements, and enzymes can potentially improve performance, recovery, and overall well-being in athletes. The use of these substances usually complements a balanced diet.

Ginseng, for example, is a traditional herb reputed for its energizing properties. Athletes might use it to enhance stamina and physical endurance. Similarly, turmeric, resveratrol, and tart cherry juice have been shown to exhibit anti-inflammatory properties, which can help with recovery and injury prevention.

However, athletes need to be careful about the usage of herbs and supplements. Not everything that is natural is safe or effective, and some substances might have side effects or interact negatively with other medications. It's crucial to consult with a knowledgeable healthcare professional before starting any new regimen.

5.4. Dietary Considerations

Nutrition plays a significant role in enhancing athletic performance. Several athletes have adopted plant-based or vegan diets as an alternative to conventional eating habits. A well-planned plant-based diet can provide all of the necessary nutrients needed for peak performance.

Plant-based diets are high in carbohydrates, the primary source of energy for athletes, and rich in antioxidants which aid recovery. Athletes following a plant-based diet need to plan well to ensure they get adequate protein, essential fats, vitamins, and minerals.

While the discussed methods are becoming increasingly popular among athletes, it is important to remember that what may work for one person might not work for another. A comprehensive approach that combines traditional and alternative therapies tailored for each individual is usually the best for optimal performance, recovery, and overall health. Athletes must maintain an open dialogue with their healthcare providers and ensure they are informed about the potential risks and benefits associated with each treatment approach.

Chapter 6. Vegetarian and Vegan Lifestyles in Athletes

Plant-based diets, namely vegetarian and vegan lifestyles, have increasingly drawn attention in the realm of sports nutrition. As athletes constantly seek new ways to optimize their performance, many have begun to recognize the potential benefits plant-based diets may offer in terms of energy, recovery, and overall health.

6.1. Advantages for Athletes

There are several potential advantages for athletes who adopt a vegetarian or vegan diet. Fueling workout routines with plant-based foods can provide the body with abundant and diverse nutrients. These diets are rich in antioxidants – substances that can help reduce inflammation and speed up recovery time. Additionally, plant-based diets are typically high in fiber, which can aid in maintaining good health and optimal weight.

It's worth noting that a well-planned vegetarian or vegan diet can meet all of an athlete's nutritional needs, including protein, which is essential for muscle development and repair. There are numerous plant-based sources of protein including legumes, whole grains, nuts, seeds, and certain vegetables. Some athletes even report increased energy levels and better performance measures after shifting to a plant-based diet.

6.2. Switching to a Plant-Based Diet

Switching to a vegetarian or vegan dietary pattern can be a significant change for many athletes. It calls for expanding one's understanding of nutrition, and making mindful and informed food choices.

When embracing plant-based diets, athletes must ensure they meet all of their dietary needs. Specifically, they should pay heed to the intake of specific nutrients which are commonly found in animal products such as iron, calcium, vitamin D, vitamin B12, and omega-3 fatty acids. All these nutrients, once predominately sourced from animal products, can be derived from plant-based sources as well.

6.3. Nutrient Requirements for Vegetarian and Vegan Athletes

The nutritional requirements of vegetarian and vegan athletes are largely similar to those of their omnivorous counterparts. However, due to the absence of animal products in their diet, there can be some exceptions.

Adequate protein consumption is paramount. While there is a common misconception that vegans and vegetarians don't get enough protein, many plant-based proteins can easily satisfy an athlete's protein need. These include foods such as lentils, chickpeas, black beans, quinoa, tofu, tempeh, and edamame, among others.

Iron is another crucial nutrient for athletes. It plays a central role in transporting oxygen throughout the body, which in turn supports athletic performance. Leafy greens, legumes, whole grains, and fortified foods can be excellent sources of iron for vegetarians and vegans.

The same attention is required to ensure adequate consumption of vitamin B12, calcium, iodine, and omega-3 fatty acids. All these nutrients are essential for an athlete's health and performance, and there are a variety of plant-based sources and supplements available to meet these needs.

6.4. Planning for Success

Successful adherence to a vegetarian or vegan lifestyle requires careful planning and knowledge about nutrition. Athletes should be aware of what their bodies need to perform and recover well, and consequently, choose foods that will provide these required nutrients.

Meal planning and preparation can play a big role in ensuring dietary needs are being met. Cooking in bulk, making use of frozen fruits and vegetables, and having suitable snacks on hand can all help in staying on track.

In all, a vegetarian or vegan diet can fuel athletic performance effectively and provide numerous health benefits. Athletes around the world, including elite-level competitors, are testament to this. However, athletes interested in making the switch should consider seeking advice from a registered dietitian or nutrition professional familiar with plant-based diets. With careful planning and a few adjustments, athletes can meet all of their nutritional needs with plant-based foods, potentially improve recovery times, and possibly even enhance performance.

Chapter 7. Yoga and Mindfulness for Improved Stamina

Yoga and mindfulness, two ancient disciplines steeped in centuries of tradition, have recently gained global recognition due to their broad applicability and numerous health benefits. By incorporating these practices into their regimen, athletes can significantly improve their stamina and overall performance.

7.1. Understanding Yoga

Yoga, rooted in ancient Indian philosophy, is an integrative mind-body practice aiming to establish mental, physical, and spiritual equilibrium. Comprising various postures (asanas), breathing techniques (pranayama), and meditation (dhyana), it facilitates a fine balance between strength, flexibility, and mindful awareness.

Yoga is a powerful tool to enhance athletic stamina because it strengthens critical muscle groups, augments flexibility, and, remarkably, strengthens the body's internal mechanisms, including the respiratory and cardiovascular systems. These physiological benefits, coupled with mindful practice, lead to significant improvements in stamina, endurance, and athletic performance.

7.2. Yoga's Impact on Physical Stamina

Yoga directly helps build physical stamina by targeting specific muscle groups. The variety of asanas practiced in yoga sessions can be adjusted to target various body parts, such as the core, legs, and upper body. Incorporating the right combination of asanas in one's routine can help develop strength and endurance in these areas.

For example, the Warrior Pose series targets the lower body, strengthens the thighs, and builds endurance. Plank and Boat Poses enhance core strength, a critical component for any sport. Enhanced muscular strength and endurance contribute to robust physical stamina in athletes.

7.3. Yogic Breathing for Stamina Enhancement

Yogic breathing techniques, known as Pranayama, play a pivotal role in augmenting an athletes' cardiovascular capacity; in turn, improving stamina. By training and practicing slow, deep, and mindful breathing, athletes can increase their lung capacity, thereby enhancing the efficiency of oxygen intake and carbon dioxide expulsion.

Pranayama like Kapalabhati (Skull-Shining Breath) and Bhastrika (Bellows Breath), when practiced regularly, boost lung function and encourage more effective oxygen utilization in the body. Both processes are crucial for improving stamina as better oxygenation directly influences energy generation in the body.

7.4. Yoga for Flexibility and Injury Prevention

Enhanced flexibility is a key benefit of yoga that directly impacts stamina and overall performance. Increased flexibility results in a broader range of motion, which can enhance the efficiency of movements and reduce the energy required for certain actions. This improved efficiency can lead to better stamina.

Moreover, regular yoga reduces the risk of injuries by improving the body's flexibility and strength. Soft tissues like muscles, ligaments, and tendons become more durable and less prone to damage, keeping athletes healthier and in the game for longer periods.

7.5. Understanding Mindfulness

Mindfulness refers to the practice of focusing one's awareness on the present moment, acknowledging and accepting feelings, thoughts, and bodily sensations without judgment. It is a mental state achieved by meditation, and it encourages self-awareness, focused attention, and a non-reactive mindset.

7.6. Mindfulness and Athletic Performance

Mindfulness can significantly influence athletic performance, including stamina and endurance. Mindful athletes tend to have greater focus, better stress management, and improved pain tolerance, which are all factors that contribute to enhanced stamina and enduring performance.

Meditation, Guided Imagery, and Body Scan techniques among other mindfulness exercises help in achieving mental clarity and focus, allowing athletes to "stay in the zone" during their performance. The practice of mindfulness develops emotional resilience which helps in overcoming performance-related anxiety and stress, ultimately aiding stamina over a long-term period.

7.7. Enhanced Pain Tolerance

Regular practice of mindfulness can increase an athlete's pain tolerance, indirectly affecting endurance levels. The ability to acknowledge discomfort without reacting and maintaining focus despite physical discomfort can help an athlete push beyond their apparent limits. This mental fortitude is vital for creating and sustaining high levels of stamina.

In conclusion, integrating yoga and mindfulness into one's fitness regimen can yield broad benefits for stamina and overall athletic performance. By fostering physical strength, flexibility, efficient breathing, mental resilience, focus, and pain tolerance, these practices can prove to be a game-changer for athletes looking to raise their performance benchmarks.

Athletes looking to incorporate these practices into their routine should gradually start with beginner-level postures and techniques, ideally under professional guidance, progressing steadily towards more complex asanas and mindfulness exercises. Always remember, just like physical training, yoga and mindfulness also require patience, consistency, and discipline – the rewards of which are worth the effort.

Chapter 8. Acupuncture: Redefining Injury Management

Acupuncture, a traditional Chinese medical practice, was cultivated more than 2,500 years ago. However, its potential benefits to athletes and how it's being utilized in the management of sports injuries are comparatively more recent developments.

8.1. Basics of Acupuncture

Acupuncture involves the insertion of thin needles into the body at particular points, known as acupoints, to stimulate various physiological responses. There are 361 acupoints in the human body, each interconnected with different organs and bodily functions. The basic idea is that health is maintained by the balanced flow of Qi (pronounced 'Chee'), or life energy, within the body. Disease or disorder, including physical injuries, are a result of an imbalance or blockage of this energy flow.

The treatment's goal is to help restore that balance, promoting self-healing. When an acupuncture needle is inserted, it stimulates sensory nerves under the skin and in the muscles resulting in the body producing natural substances, such as pain-relieving endorphins. It's likely these naturally released substances are responsible for the beneficial effects of acupuncture.

8.2. Acupuncture in Sports Medicine

In conventional Western medicine, acupuncture has been increasingly integrated into orthopedics and sports medicine. Various studies indicate acupuncture could help reduce inflammation, improve circulation, relieve muscle spasm, and speed up healing of soft tissue injuries, making it a practical strategy for injury management.

Given the growing demand for non-drug interventions among athletes and active individuals, acupuncture proves to be an attractive choice. Many common sports injuries, such as sprains, strains, pulled muscles, shin splints, and even tennis elbow or golfer's elbow can be effectively managed through acupuncture therapy.

The use of acupuncture for the resolution of acute injuries is straightforward and generally well accepted. Certain acupoints have demonstrated effectiveness in treating specific types of injuries and pain, and these points are regularly used in treatments. Acupuncturists generally offer treatments on the sidelines of games and martial arts tournaments to assist in immediate injury relief.

8.3. Immediate Impact of Acupuncture on Injuries

Acupuncture has a few immediate benefits when used for sports injuries. Treatment at the site of the injury helps to reduce pain and inflammation. It can also resolve bruising by increasing local circulation, dissipating the bruising and quicken the healing process.

In contrast, whole-body treatment can help improve overall performance by increasing energy, improving sleep, reducing stress, and giving a sense of total well-being, thus creating a healthier environment within which the body can heal itself. This dual approach to treatment can enhance both the resolution of the immediate injury and the function and health of the athlete in general.

8.4. Acupuncture and Pain Relief

One of the major benefits of incorporating acupuncture into injury treatment plans is its analgesic, or pain-relieving, effect. It is believed that acupuncture affects the spinal cord's pain-processing centers, decreasing their activity and lowering pain thresholds.

Acupuncture treatments also stimulate blood flow. This increase in blood flow brings fresh oxygen, nutrients, and immune cells to the injured area to begin the repair process. On the flip side, the enhanced circulation removes waste products and inflammatory compounds, speeding up tissue recovery.

Studies suggest that acupuncture can have a significant impact on specific kinds of chronic pain, including lower back pain, osteoarthritis pain, and even severe headaches or migraines. These effects of acupuncture bring potential benefits to athletes suffering from these chronic conditions.

8.5. The Role of Acupuncture in Injury Rehabilitation

Rehabilitation is a key concern for any athlete coming off an injury. Here too, acupuncture can play a crucial part. Therapists can use it to facilitate muscle recovery while also ensuring that the connective tissue heals correctly. Acupuncture can also help to control pain during this recovery process following intense physical therapy sessions.

In addition, acupuncture can assist with the mental and emotional aspects of long-term injury recovery. The stimulation of specific acupoints can help to relieve symptoms of anxiety and depression associated with long periods away from training or competition.

8.6. Limitations of Acupuncture in Sports and Injury Management

Invariably, while acupuncture provides numerous benefits, it is also important to note that it hardly replaces all conventional Western methods and treatments. The impact varies from person to person, with two individuals receiving the same treatment for similar injuries experiencing different outcomes. As such, acupuncture should not be considered a magic bullet but instead a potential part of a comprehensive treatment strategy.

Moreover, the quality and experience of the acupuncturist greatly impact the outcome of the treatment, hence, selecting a qualified, experienced practitioner is crucial.

In conclusion, acupuncture is a fascinating and growing field within sports medicine with significant therapeutic potential. From initial injury treatment, pain relief to rehabilitation, acupuncture offers a complementary path for holistic injury management for athletes. Future research will further optimize its use, enhancing our understanding of best practices and integration with other treatments for maximum effect. Its relevance is only projected to increase as athletes continue to seek safe, effective, and natural methods to increase performance and maintain health.

Chapter 9. Natural Supplements: Boosting Performance Holistically

Natural Supplements offer an incredible array of health-boosting properties, particularly for athletes who are constantly striving to enhance their performance. Turning to nature for nourishment can be a transformative choice, leading to improved strength, faster recovery, and optimized overall health.

9.1. The Role of Natural Supplements in Performance Enhancement

All athlete's mission to perform better is a multi-faceted process that involves strengthening the body, boosting endurance, improving recovery times, and maintaining general health. Traditionally, many rely on synthetic enhancements to gain that competitive edge. However, with an increased understanding of our individual health dynamics, there's been a shift toward natural supplements. Natural supplements, derived from food or plant sources, can provide the body with essential nutrients missing from one's diet. They have lower chances of causing adverse side-effects and are often easy to incorporate into daily routines.

9.2. Popular Natural Supplements for Athletes

There's a wide range of natural sports supplements available, each with their specific advantages. Here are a few that have gained significant recognition:

- *Beta-Alanine*: An amino acid that aids muscle endurance during high-intensity workouts. It works by buffering the lactic acid in muscles, delaying fatigue and enabling longer workouts.

- *Branched-Chain Amino Acids (BCAAs)*: These include leucine, isoleucine, and valine. BCAAs assist in muscle recovery and help reduce muscle soreness post-exercise.

- *Creatine*: Synthesized by the body and found in meat and fish, creatine provides muscles with the energy needed for high-intensity, short-duration exercise.

- *Turmeric*: Curcumin, the active constituent of turmeric, is a potent anti-inflammatory and antioxidant agent and can help heal and recover the body's systems post-workout.

9.3. Comprehensive Benefits of Natural Supplements

Natural supplements, unlike synthetic ones, have benefits spanning beyond athletic performance. Some of the broader benefits include:

- *Reduced Inflammation*: Many athletic injuries and pains are due to inflammation. Natural supplements like turmeric and omega-3 fatty acids have powerful anti-inflammatory properties.

- *Improved Cardiovascular Health*: Substances like Coenzyme Q10 and Omega-3 fatty acids can contribute to a healthier heart and improved cardiovascular function.

- *Enhanced Immunity*: Athletes need a robust immune system. Vitamins A, C, and E, along with minerals like zinc, can bolster the body's natural defenses.

- *Promotion of Overall Well-being*: Supplements like adaptogenic herbs supports the body's response to stress, promoting an overall sense of well-being, which indirectly impacts athletic performance.

9.4. Sourcing and Consumption of Natural Supplements

Natural supplements can be taken in various forms, including tablets, capsules, powders, teas, and tinctures. It is advisable to consult with a healthcare provider or a certified nutritionist before beginning any supplement regimen. Quality and sourcing are of utmost importance when choosing natural supplements. Prioritize obtaining them from reputable sellers.

9.5. Cutting Through the Hype: Realities vs Expectations

While the benefits of natural supplements are many, it's essential to maintain a realistic outlook. Supplements can support fitness goals, but they are not a substitute for a balanced diet, proper training, and adequate rest. They serve as an augmenting element in an athlete's fitness journey, rather than an all-encompassing solution.

9.6. The Future: Personalized Supplementation

One size does not fit all when it comes to nutrition and supplementation. The future may lie in personalized supplementation, tailored according to individual needs, lifestyles, and genetic predispositions. Advancements in scientific research are heading towards more individualized supplement strategies that consider athletes' metabolism, body composition, gut microbiota, and more.

Embracing natural supplements could potentially form an integral part of your holistic fitness journey, intricately intertwined with optimal nutrition and exercise. Consider your athletic goals, current health, lifestyle habits, and consult the proper professionals to aid in stewarding your holistic journey to peak performance.

Chapter 10. Sports Psychology: A Holistic Assessment

Sports psychology often carries a one-dimensional perspective, primarily focused on optimizing mental performance. Yet, holistic sports psychology broadens this perspective, taking into account emotional, physical, and spiritual factors to produce not just a high-performing athlete but a healthier, more fulfilled one. The following will delve into key areas of holistic sports psychology, offering techniques, assessments, and discussions that may enhance wellbeing and performance in tandem.

10.1. The Interplay of Mind, Body, and Spirit

Holistic sports psychology recognizes the interconnectivity of mental, physical, and spiritual aspects in athletic performance. It promotes the idea that an individual's psychological state can influence their physical health and vice versa, while their spiritual beliefs and practices can enhance wellbeing and resilience.

Several techniques may facilitate harmony between these aspects. For example, athletes can employ mindfulness, a mental state achieved by focusing awareness on the present moment while calmly acknowledging and accepting feelings, thoughts, and bodily sensation. Regular mindfulness practice can have significant psychological benefits, providing a powerful tool for managing stress, improving focus, and enhancing emotional intelligence.

10.2. Nutrition and Holistic Health

An essential aspect of holistic health is the understanding that nutrition significantly impacts mental and physical health. Consuming a balanced diet ensures the body and brain receive the necessary nutrients to function optimally and can influence mood and energy levels, critical for athletic performance.

Research continually emphasizes the mental benefits of consuming various nutrients. For example, Omega-3 fatty acids, found in fatty fish and some seeds and nuts, have been linked to improvements in mood and cognitive function. Additionally, the gut-brain connection, a hot topic in recent health discussions, highlights the impact of gut health on mental wellbeing, further solidifying the importance of nutrition in sports psychology.

10.3. Holistic Techniques for Stress and Injury Management

Stress and injuries are inevitable realities for athletes. Holistic sports psychology offers unique approaches to manage them, by incorporating both traditional psychological interventions and alternative therapies.

One primary focus of this approach is fostering mental resilience. Techniques like cognitive-behavioral therapy (CBT) can help athletes develop healthy thinking habits and resilience in face of adversity. Furthermore, approaches like guided imagery and hypnosis can facilitate pain management and speed up injury recovery.

Alternative therapies can augment these techniques. For instance, acupuncture can release muscle tension and promote healing, while mindfulness-based stress reduction strategies can aid in stress management and improve mental clarity.

10.4. Spirituality in Sports

The role of spirituality in sports generally gets limited attention. But in holistic sports psychology, it's recognized as a key contributing influence on both performance and wellbeing. Athletes can draw strength, motivation, and resilience from their spiritual beliefs, while practices like yoga promote flexibility, mindfulness, and self-awareness.

Though 'spirituality' carries different meanings for different individuals, fostering a deeper sense of meaning, purpose, or connection can greatly enhance motivation, resilience, and overall happiness, thereby boosting performance.

10.5. The Psychology of Holistic Practices

Lastly, understanding the psychology behind holistic techniques can empower athletes to use them more effectively. Mental rehearsal—envisioning a successful performance—can help 'program' the body to perform optimally under pressure. Biofeedback—where athletes can learn to control certain physical processes, such as heart rate—promotes self-awareness, aiding mental and physical regulation during performance.

Holistic sports psychology enables athletes to comprehend and influence the interplay between their mental, physical, and spiritual aspects, facilitating improved performance and wellbeing. By incorporating balanced nutrition, mental resilience techniques, stress and injury management, spirituality, plus an understanding of the psychology behind these practices, athletes can be empowered to reach new heights in their athletic pursuits, and more importantly—find greater enjoyment in doing so.

Chapter 11. Creating a Personalized Holistic Athletic Plan

A holistic approach to athletic training is a comprehensive method to fitness that harmonizes the mind and body with your lifestyle choices, effectively integrating various other elements into your regimen. Whilst reaching for your prime physical performance, you should also foster the health of your mind and soul to accomplish an overall wellbeing. This chapter will guide you on creating a personalized holistic athletic plan, tailored to your unique needs and specifications.

11.1. Establishing Your Fitness Goals

Before crafting a personalized plan, outlining your fitness goals is crucial. These directives should be specific, measurable, attainable, relevant and time-based (the SMART approach). This entails being completely realistic about your expectations and what you hope to achieve within a certain timeframe.

Goal setting expands beyond physical targets. Mental health such as reducing stress and having a positive mindset, along with dietary changes and personal development opportunities, can be factored in. Always reassess your goals, this helps to visualize the progression and stimulate motivation.

11.2. Understanding Your Current Fitness and Health Level

Taking account of your current fitness level is critical before you begin any program. Gauge your cardiovascular fitness, strength, flexibility and body composition. You will also want to give thought to potential health issues that could affect your ability to exercise. If needed, get a full medical examination to ensure any underlying health issues are detected early.

11.3. Incorporating Calmness and Mindfulness

Mindfulness and calmness are crucial components of a rounded holistic athletic plan. Techniques such as yoga and meditation can be instrumental in reducing stress, boosting your mood, and improving your focus and mental fitness, all of which contribute significantly to your physical performance.

11.4. Nutrition and Dietary Guidelines

The foods you eat will significantly influence your performance. Adequate nourishment can enhance your recovery and energy levels, bolster your immune system, and provide the necessary fuel for workouts. Tailoring your food intake according to your nutritional requirements and goals should be incorporated.

Ensure to consume wholesome foods, abundant in fruits, vegetables, lean proteins, and whole grains. Remember, hydration is equally as important, and you need to drink ample fluids especially if you're exercising rigorously.

11.5. Choosing Your Preferred Exercise Modalities

The type of exercise should align with your fitness goals and individual preferences. You might engage in cardiovascular activities like running, cycling, or swimming, strength training, flexibility exercises, or a mix of these.

Refresh your workout routines occasionally to prevent monotony and fitness plateaus. Each form of exercise comes with its own set of benefits. Choosing a variety that you enjoy can enhance your commitment and improve overall health.

11.6. Recovery and Rest

Rest and recovery are often overlooked but are essential. Proper recovery allows your body to heal, preventing injuries and allowing you to train more effectively. Sleep, in particular, plays a crucial role in the recovery process and should not be underestimated.

11.7. Alternative Therapies and Supplements

Consider incorporating alternative therapies such as chiropractic, acupuncture, or massage into your holistic plan. These may aid in injury prevention and recovery and improve your wellness quotient.

Many athletes use supplementation to enhance performance. However, always consult with a specialist before adopting any new supplements to thwart any adverse effects.

11.8. Monitoring Progress and Adjusting the Plan

Regularly checking on your progress is significant. Set periodic benchmarks and evaluate your performance against these. Recognize when adjustments are needed. If you hit a plateau, do not hesitate to modify your plan and introduce new elements.

Remember, the journey to holistic fitness is a marathon, not a sprint. Be patient with yourself and have a positive mindset. With dedication and consistency, you're sure to see substantial progress in your overall health and athletic performance.

www.ingramcontent.com/pod-product-compliance
Lightning Source LLC
Chambersburg PA
CBHW060853260726
48661CB00008B/3242